No Gallbladder Diet Cookbook for Seniors

A Nourishing Guide to Long-Term Wellness after Gallbladder Removal Surgery - Quick and Easy, Flavorful Low-Fat Recipes for Effortless Digestion

+Bonus 1: 21-day meal plan for no gall bladder diet

+Bonus 2: Over 10 pages of meal planner journal

DR. Kimberly Thorpe

Copyright © [2024] by DR. Kimberly Thorpe

About the author

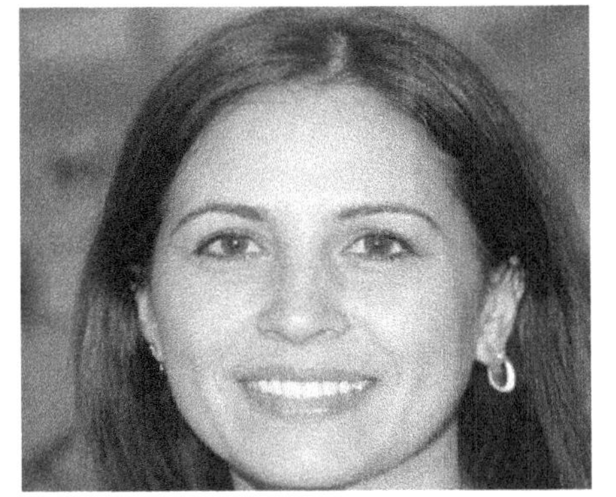

Dr. Kimberly Thorpe is not only a seasoned dietitian and nutritionist but also a dedicated advocate for holistic health and wellness. With a profound passion for empowering individuals to heal themselves and achieve their fullest potential, Dr. Thorpe has become a guiding force in the field of health and self-improvement.

With a wealth of experience in the realm of nutrition, Dr. Thorpe has authored several acclaimed health cookbooks and self-help books. Her works delve into the intersection of nutrition, lifestyle, and overall well-being, offering readers practical insights and guidance on their journey to a healthier and more balanced life.

Beyond her professional endeavors, Dr. Kimberly Thorpe is a devoted mother of two, cherishing the joys of family life. Her commitment to holistic health extends beyond the pages of her books, as she practices what she preaches, fostering a balanced and mindful lifestyle.

Dr. Thorpe's writing is infused with a genuine desire to inspire positive change, drawing on her expertise to guide readers toward healthier choices. Her holistic approach emphasizes the interconnectedness of mind, body, and spirit, reflecting a belief in the transformative power of self-care and self-discovery.

As a sought-after speaker and educator, Dr. Kimberly Thorpe continues to share her knowledge and passion with audiences around the world. Her mission is to create a ripple effect of wellness, encouraging individuals to embrace their unique journey toward a more vibrant and fulfilling life.

In her downtime, Dr. Thorpe enjoys nothing more than spending quality time with her family, finding joy in simple pleasures and creating lasting memories. Through her writing and personal example, she invites readers to join her on the path to holistic well-being and to discover the transformative potential within themselves.

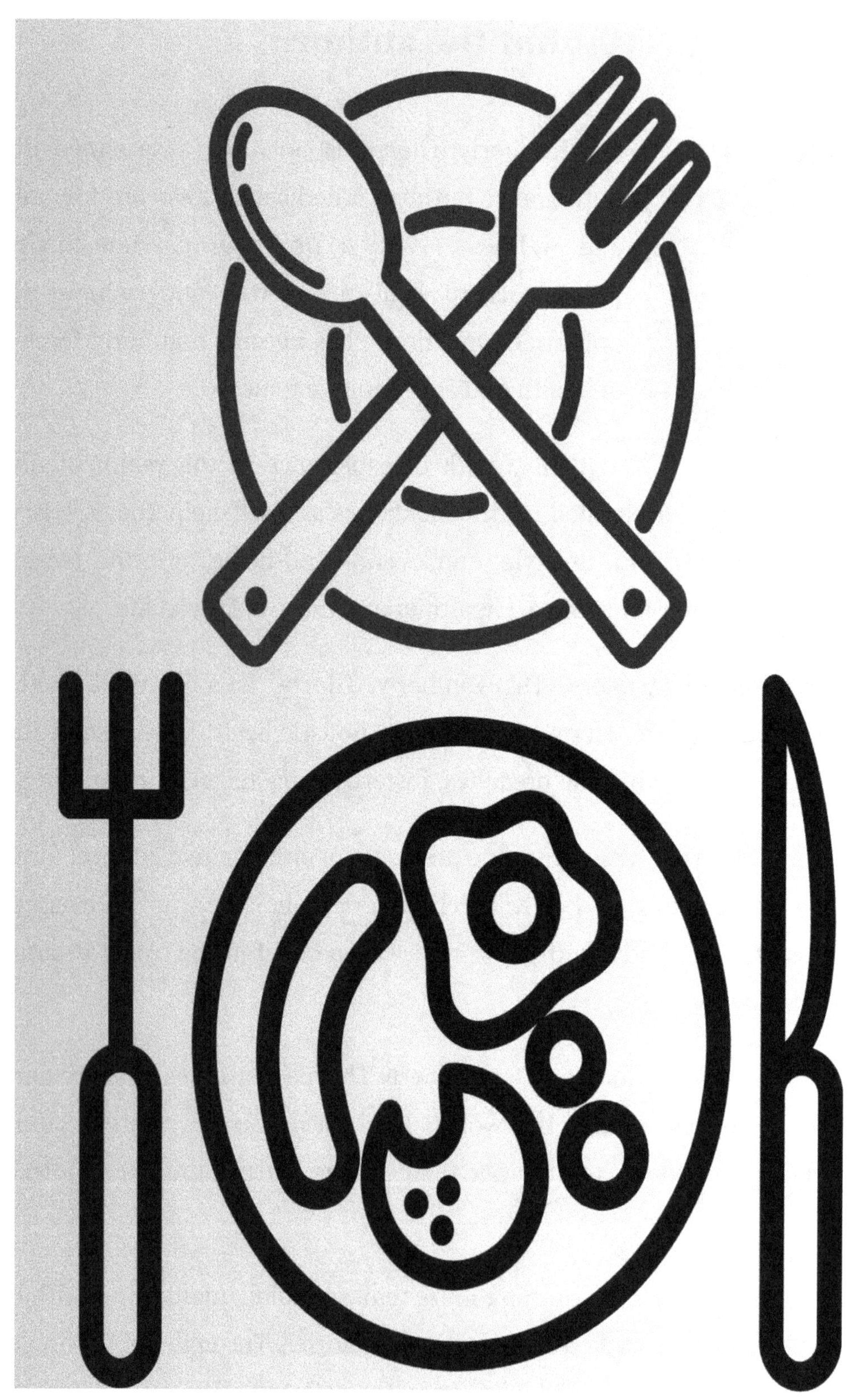

Table of contents

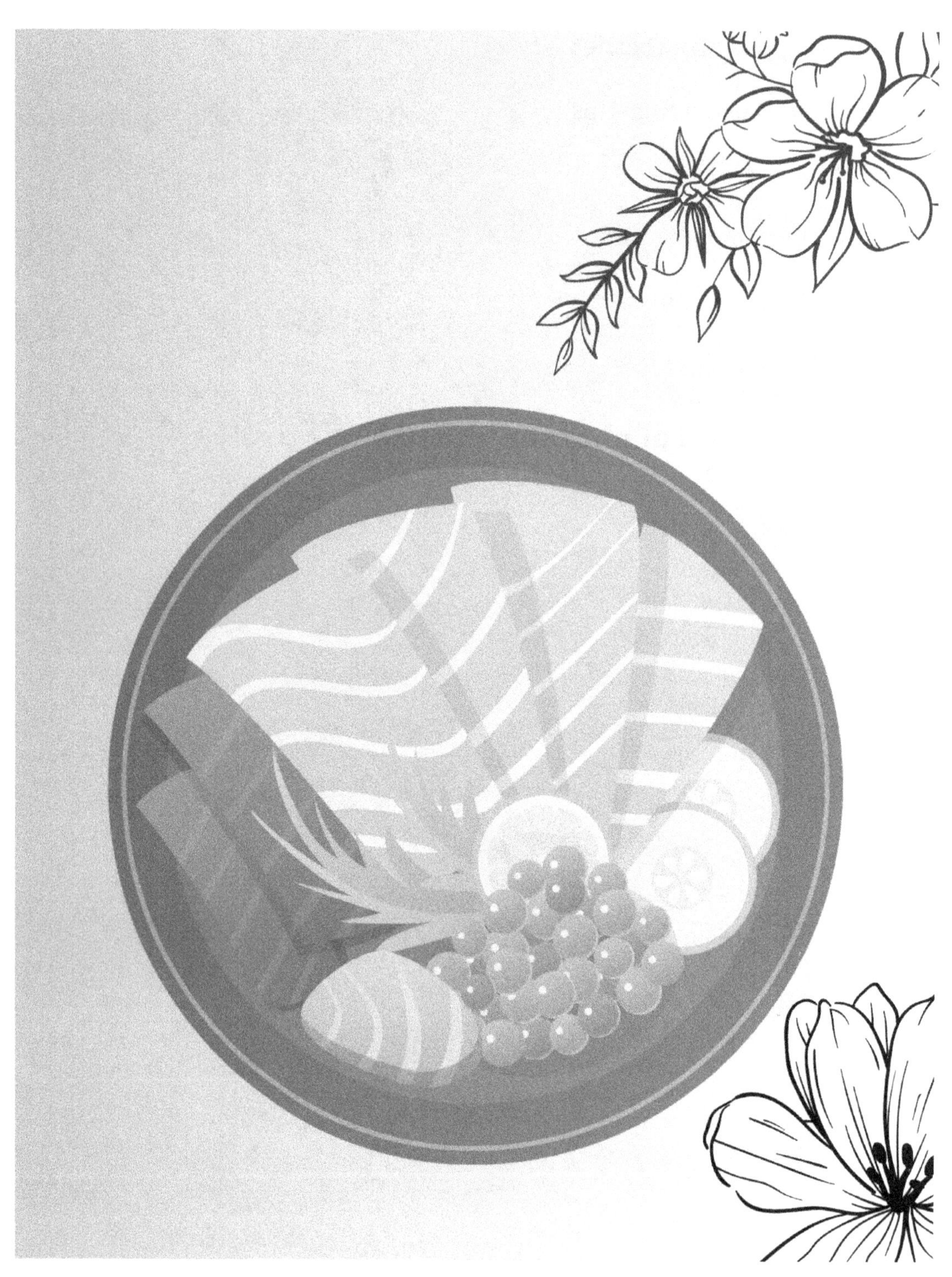

Introduction

Meet Evelyn, a vivacious and insightful person who has stayed resilient and enthusiastic in the face of adversity. Her path to a no-gallbladder diet began when she understood the transformational potential of good eating. The simple process of selecting nutrient-dense foods became not only a daily ritual, but also a catalyst for fresh vitality.

Evelyn's story is not uncommon; it reflects the experiences of many seniors who have gone on a similar journey for happiness. As we explore the world of the "No Gallbladder Diet Cookbook for Seniors," we start on a trip driven by the conviction that a healthy diet is more than simply a choice, but a powerful instrument that can impact how we experience life in our golden years.

This cookbook is more than just a compilation of dishes; it's a guide to intestinal harmony. I welcome you to peruse the pages that follow, which are loaded with culinary delicacies carefully prepared to nurture both body and spirit. Each meal exemplifies the idea that excellent food is about more than simply nourishment; it's about relishing the tastes of life and embracing the joy that comes with taking control of our health.

So, let this cookbook serve as your guide, providing not only tasty dishes geared toward seniors, but also a road map to a more vibrant and fulfilling existence. Remember that every bite is a step toward well-being, and every chapter is a celebration of the amazing adventure that is life as you embark on this gourmet trip.

Brief overview of gallbladder function and the impact of its removal on digestion.

The gallbladder is a tiny organ found beneath the liver that stores and concentrates bile produced by the liver. Bile is essential for fat breakdown and absorption in the small intestine.

When we eat a fat-containing meal, the gallbladder releases bile into the digestive tract, which aids in the breakdown of lipids into smaller particles that are more easily absorbed by the body.

The storage and concentration of bile are altered when the gallbladder is removed, a process known as cholecystectomy. This surgical procedure is frequently required due to gallstones, inflammation, or other gallbladder-related disorders. While the body can still create bile in the absence of the gallbladder, the digestion process can be affected.

The continual leak of bile into the small intestine is eliminated when the gallbladder is removed. As a result, there may be a diminished ability to emulsify and absorb dietary lipids. This alteration can cause problems with fat absorption, leading in symptoms like bloating, gas, and diarrhea, especially after eating high-fat meals.

Individuals who have had their gallbladders removed may benefit from a modified diet to accommodate these changes in digestion. This frequently entails limiting high-fat diets and introducing readily digestible options to reduce digestive discomfort and enhance general well-being. The "No Gallbladder Diet Cookbook for Seniors" is intended to address these dietary changes, offering dishes and advice targeted to the specific needs of seniors who have had their gallbladder removed.

Benefits of the No Gallbladder Diet for Seniors

The "No Gallbladder Diet" provides various advantages to people who have had their gallbladder removed. Here are some significant benefits:

1. Improved Digestive Comfort: Following a no gallbladder diet might help decrease digestive discomfort, such as bloating, gas, and diarrhea, which can occur as a result of changes in fat digestion.

2. *Reduced Risk of Dietary disorders:* Because the gallbladder is in charge of storing and releasing bile to aid in fat digestion, a modified diet can lower the risk of dietary disorders that may emerge when fats are not properly processed.

3. *Balanced Fat Intake:* The diet encourages a balanced approach to fat consumption, emphasizing good fats while minimizing saturated and trans fat intake. This can help with overall heart health.

4. *Promotes Nutrient Absorption:* The no gallbladder diet promotes the absorption of key fat-soluble vitamins such as A, D, E, and K by consuming nutrient-dense foods and optimizing fat digestion.

5. *Weight Management:* The diet promotes the intake of nutrient-rich, whole foods over high-fat processed choices, which may help with weight management.

6. *Maintaining Consistent Blood Sugar Levels:* Eating complex carbohydrates, fiber, and lean proteins will help keep blood sugar levels stable, promoting overall energy and well-being.

7. *Improved Bowel Regularity:* Adopting a fiber-rich, readily digestible diet can help with bowel regularity, reducing the likelihood of constipation or irregular bowel movements.

8. Elders' Customization: The "No Gallbladder Diet Cookbook for Seniors" specially tailors meals to the individual needs and preferences of elders, guaranteeing that dietary changes are both helpful and enjoyable.

9. *Encourages a Healthier Lifestyle:* A no-gallbladder diet frequently corresponds with wider concepts of a healthy lifestyle, encouraging seniors to make conscious eating choices and emphasize their overall well-being.

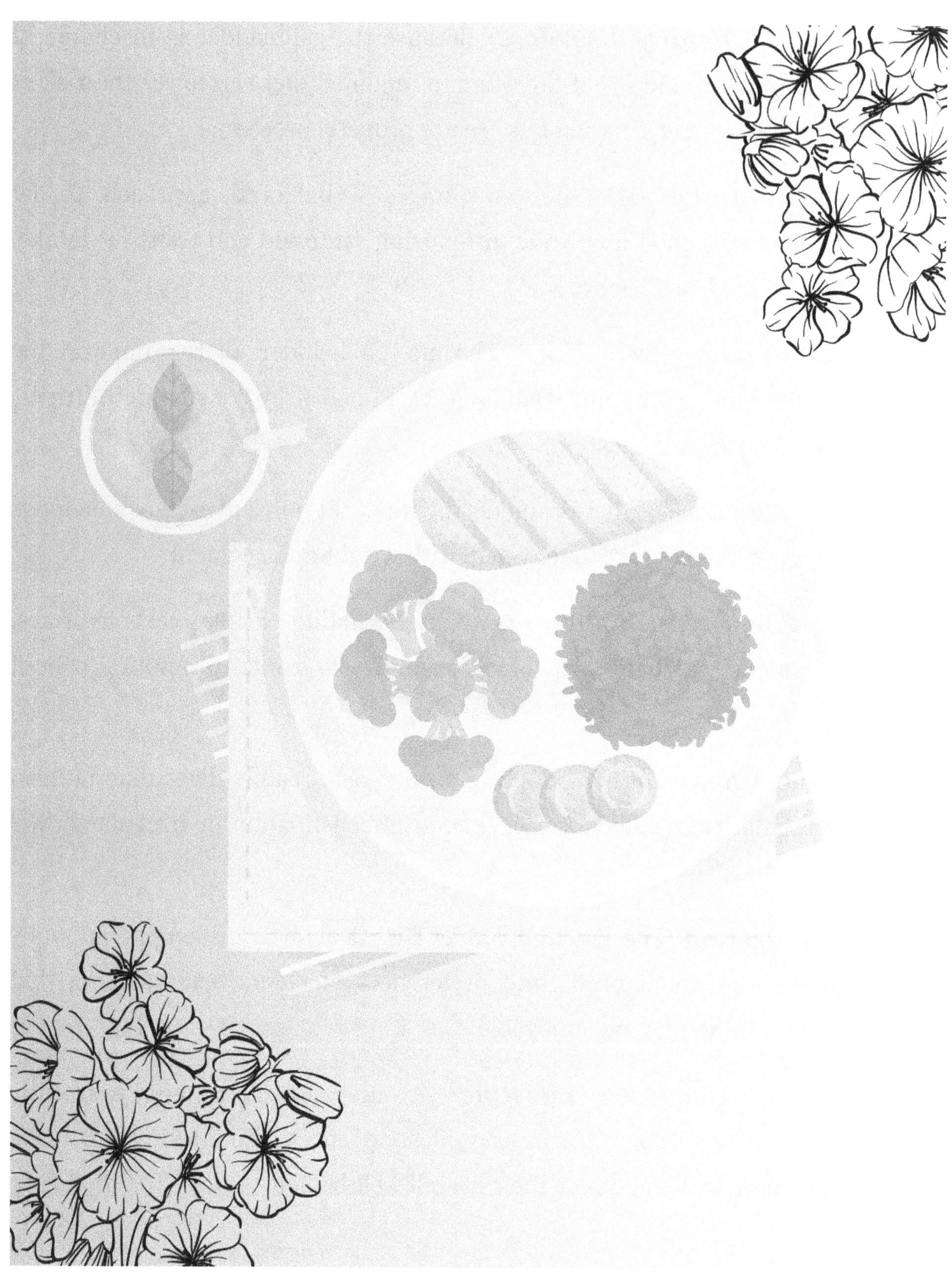

Common challenges faced by seniors after gallbladder removal

Seniors may face a variety of hurdles following gallbladder removal, as the loss of this organ can impair digestion and cause unique problems. The following are some of the most common issues that seniors confront following gallbladder removal:

1. Trouble Digesting Fats: The gallbladder contains bile, which aids in fat digestion. Without the gallbladder, seniors may have difficulty adequately breaking down and absorbing dietary lipids, resulting in symptoms such as bloating, gas, and diarrhea.

2. Food Sensitivity: Seniors may acquire an increased sensitivity to high-fat or fatty foods, which can cause stomach pain. Certain foods that were previously accepted may now cause problems due to changes in fat digestion.

3. Meal-Related pain: Seniors may endure pain and bloating, especially after high-fat meals. This can affect their pleasure of food and cause them to avoid specific foods.

4. Concerns about Nutrient Absorption: The gallbladder is involved in the absorption of fat-soluble vitamins (A, D, E, and K). Seniors may have difficulty absorbing these critical minerals, thus affecting their general health and well-being.

5. Unpredictable Bowel Movements: The loss of the gallbladder can cause bowel patterns to shift, including diarrhea. Seniors may endure erratic bowel motions, which can disrupt their regular routines and cause discomfort.

6. Adaptation to Dietary Changes: For seniors, adjusting to a modified diet that accommodates changes in fat digestion can be difficult; they may need to make considerable modifications to their eating patterns, which can be both physically and emotionally taxing.

7. *Impact on Lifestyle and Social Eating:* Seniors may discover that their dietary limitations limit their capacity to participate in food-related social activities. This can result in emotions of loneliness and dissatisfaction.

8. *Weight Management Difficulties:* Some seniors may have difficulty managing their weight following gallbladder ectomy. Changes in fat digestion may affect calorie absorption and overall nutritional intake.

9. *Potential Gastrointestinal Symptoms:* As a result of changes in digestion following gallbladder removal, seniors may have gastrointestinal symptoms such as indigestion, abdominal discomfort, or a feeling of fullness.

10. *Dietary help:* Many seniors may want assistance and help in navigating their dietary demands following gallbladder ectomy. Seeking help from healthcare specialists or licensed dietitians can be quite beneficial in dealing with these issues.

The fundamentals of transitioning to a no-gallbladder diet.

Making smart dietary choices to manage digestion successfully is required when adapting to a no gallbladder diet. Here are some general principles to help people make this transition:

1. *Slowly Reintroduce Fats:* Begin by gradually reinstating fats into the diet in lesser amounts. This permits the body to adjust to the alterations in fat digestion that occur after the gallbladder is removed.

2. *Choose Healthy Fats:* Choose healthy fats like avocados, olive oil, almonds, and fatty seafood. These fats are easy to digest and include important nutrients.

3. *Moderation is essential:* Consume fats sparingly to avoid overloading the digestive system. Smaller, more frequent meals may be more manageable than bigger, less frequent ones.

4. *Emphasize Lean Proteins:* Include lean protein sources in your meals such as poultry, fish, tofu, and lentils. In general, lean proteins are easier to digest and put less load on the digestive system.

5. *Select Whole Foods:* Choose whole, unprocessed foods that are high in fiber, vitamins, and minerals. These foods promote intestinal health and give critical nutrients.

6. *Mindful Eating:* Practice mindful eating by thoroughly chewing food and appreciating each bite. This helps to break down food before it enters the digestive system.

7. *Avoid High-Fat Foods:* Avoid high-fat foods, fried foods, and overly processed snacks. These can be difficult for the digestive system to process without the help of the gallbladder.

8. *Maintain Adequate hydrated:* Adequate hydrated aids digestion. Drink enough of water throughout the day to aid in the elimination of waste products and the smooth operation of the digestive system.

9. *Eat Smaller, More regular Meals:* Instead of three substantial meals per day, consider eating smaller, more regular meals throughout the day. This can assist in managing the digestive load and preventing pain.

10. *Avoid Trigger Foods:* Recognize and avoid specific foods that may cause stomach distress. Pay attention to how your body reacts to various meals and change your diet accordingly.

11. *Eat Fiber-Rich Foods:* Include fiber-rich foods like fruits, vegetables, and whole grains in your diet. Fiber improves digestion and can aid in the regulation of bowel motions.

12. *Manage Stress:* Stress might interfere with digestion. In order to enhance general digestive health, incorporate stress-management approaches such as relaxation exercises, deep breathing, or mindfulness.

13. *Consult with Healthcare specialists:* For personalized assistance, seek the advice of healthcare specialists or registered dietitians. They can make customized recommendations based on an individual's health needs and aspirations.

14. *Maintain a Food journal:* Keep a food journal to note how various meals influence your digestion. When working with healthcare specialists to optimize your nutrition, this might be a beneficial tool.

Oatmeal Delight

Egg White Veggie Scramble

Smoothie Bliss

Greek Yogurt Parfait

Avocado Toast with Poached Egg

Chia Seed Pudding

Blueberry Almond Overnight Oats

Banana Nut Muffins

Raspberry Almond Smoothie Bowl

Veggie and Feta Frittata

Oatmeal Delight

Nutritional Info || Protein **10g**, Fiber **8g**, Calories **300cal**

Prep time: 10 minutes

INGREDIENTS

- 1/2 cup rolled oats

- 1 cup almond milk

- 1/2 cup mixed berries

- 1 tablespoon chia seeds

INSTRUCTIONS

1. In a saucepan, combine rolled oats and almond milk.

2. Cook over medium heat until the oats are creamy.

3. Top with mixed berries and sprinkle chia seeds.

Egg White Veggie Scramble

Nutritional Info || Protein **20g**, Fiber **3g**, Calories **150cal**

Prep time: 15 minutes

INGREDIENTS

- 3 egg whites

- 1/2 cup diced bell peppers

- 1/4 cup diced onions

- 1/4 cup spinach

INSTRUCTIONS

1. Whisk egg whites and pour into a non-stick skillet.

2. Add bell peppers, onions, and spinach.

3. Cook until eggs are set and veggies are tender.

Smoothie Bliss

Nutritional Info || Protein **15g**, Fiber **5g**, Calories **250cal**
Prep time: 5 minutes

INGREDIENTS

- 1 banana

- 1/2 cup Greek yogurt

- 1/2 cup mixed berries

- 1 tablespoon honey

INSTRUCTIONS:

1. Blend all ingredients until smooth.

2. Pour into a glass and enjoy.

Greek Yogurt Parfait

Nutritional Info || Protein **18g**, Fiber **6g**, Calories **350cal**
Prep time: 5 minutes

INGREDIENTS

- 1 cup Greek yogurt

- 1/2 cup granola

- 1/2 cup sliced strawberries

- 1 tablespoon almond butter

INSTRUCTIONS

1. In a glass, layer Greek yogurt, granola, and strawberries.

2. Drizzle with almond butter.

Avocado Toast with Poached Egg

Nutritional Info || Protein **12g**, Fiber **8g**, Calories **250cal**
Prep time: 15 minutes

INGREDIENTS

- 1 slice whole-grain bread

- 1/2 avocado, mashed

- 1 poached egg

- Salt and pepper to taste

INSTRUCTIONS

1. Toast the bread and spread mashed avocado on top.

2. Place a poached egg on top and season with salt and pepper.

Chia Seed Pudding

Nutritional Info || Protein **6g**, Fiber **10g**, Calories **200cal**
Prep time: 5 minutes

INGREDIENTS

- 3 tablespoons chia seeds

- 1 cup almond milk

- 1/2 teaspoon vanilla extract

- 1 tablespoon maple syrup

INSTRUCTIONS

1. Mix chia seeds, almond milk, vanilla extract, and maple syrup in a bowl.

2. Refrigerate overnight.

Blueberry Almond Overnight Oats

Nutritional Info || Protein **8g**, Fiber **7g**, Calories **280cal**

Prep time: 5 minutes

INGREDIENTS

- 1/2 cup rolled oats

- 1/2 cup almond milk

- 1/4 cup blueberries

- 1 tablespoon almond slices

INSTRUCTIONS

1. Combine oats, almond milk, blueberries, and almond slices in a jar.

2. Refrigerate overnight.

Banana Nut Muffins

Nutritional Info || Protein **6g**, Fiber **4g**, Calories **180cal**

Prep time: 25 minutes

INGREDIENTS

- 1 cup whole wheat flour

- 1/2 cup oats

- 1/2 cup mashed bananas

- 1/4 cup chopped walnuts

- 1/4 cup honey

- 1/4 cup Greek yogurt

INSTRUCTIONS

1. Mix all ingredients in a bowl.

2. Spoon into muffin cups and bake at 350°F (175°C) for 15-20 minutes.

Raspberry Almond Smoothie Bowl

Nutritional Info || Protein **8g**, Fiber **10g**, Calories **300cal**

Prep time: 10 minutes

INGREDIENTS

- 1 cup frozen raspberries

- 1/2 banana

- 1/2 cup almond milk

- 2 tablespoons almond butter

INSTRUCTIONS

1. Blend raspberries, banana, almond milk, and almond butter until smooth.

2. Pour into a bowl and add toppings. (Toppings: sliced almonds, chia seeds)

Veggie and Feta Frittat

Nutritional Info || Protein **15g**, Fiber **3g**, Calories **240cal**

Prep time: 20 minutes

INGREDIENTS

- 4 eggs

- 1/2 cup diced bell peppers

- 1/4 cup diced red onions

- 1/4 cup crumbled feta cheese

-Salt and pepper to taste

INSTRUCTIONS

1. Whisk eggs and mix in bell peppers, red onions, and feta.

2. Pour into a greased oven-safe skillet and bake at 375°F (190°C) for 15-20 minutes.

Grilled Chicken Salad

Quinoa and Vegetable Bowl

Vegetable Soup with Whole Grain Crackers

Baked Salmon with Herbs

Stir-Fried Tofu and Vegetables

Mashed Sweet Potatoes

Lentil and Vegetable Stew

Quinoa Salad with Chickpeas

Turkey and Vegetable Wrap

Brown Rice Bowl with Black Beans

Grilled Chicken Salad

Nutritional Info || Protein **25g**, Fiber **4g**, Calories **300cal**
Prep time: 20 minutes

INGREDIENTS

- 4 oz grilled chicken breast

- Mixed salad greens

- Cherry tomatoes

- Cucumber slices

- Olive oil and balsamic vinegar for dressing

INSTRUCTIONS

1. Grill the chicken breast and slice it.

2. Combine with salad greens, cherry tomatoes, and cucumber slices.

3. Drizzle with olive oil and balsamic vinegar.

Quinoa and Vegetable Bowl

Nutritional Info || Protein **12g**, Fiber **8g**, Calories **350cal**
Prep time: 25 minutes

INGREDIENTS

- 1/2 cup cooked quinoa

- Steamed broccoli florets

- Sliced bell peppers

- Cherry tomatoes

- Feta cheese crumbles

INSTRUCTIONS

1. Combine cooked quinoa with steamed broccoli, sliced bell peppers, and cherry tomatoes.

2. Top with feta cheese crumbles.

Vegetable Soup with Whole Grain Crackers

Nutritional Info || Protein **4g**, Fiber **6g**, Calories **180cal**
Prep time: 30 minutes

INGREDIENTS

- 2 cups vegetable broth

- Mixed vegetables (carrots, celery, zucchini)

- 1/2 cup whole grain crackers

INSTRUCTIONS

1. Simmer mixed vegetables in vegetable broth until tender.

2. Serve with whole grain crackers on the side.

Baked Salmon with Herbs

Nutritional Info || Protein **30g**, Fiber **1g**, Calories **350cal**
Prep time: 25 minutes

INGREDIENTS

- 6 oz salmon fillet

- Fresh herbs (dill, parsley)

- Lemon slices

- Olive oil

INSTRUCTIONS

1. Season salmon with fresh herbs and lemon slices.

2. Bake at 400°F (200°C) for 15-20 minutes.

Stir-Fried Tofu and Vegetables

Nutritional Info || Protein **15g**, Fiber **6g**, Calories **250cal**
Prep time: 20 minutes

INGREDIENTS

- 1 cup tofu, cubed

- Mixed stir-fry vegetables (broccoli, bell peppers, snap peas)

- Soy sauce and ginger for seasoning

INSTRUCTIONS

1. Stir-fry tofu and mixed vegetables in a pan.

2. Season with soy sauce and ginger.

Mashed Sweet Potatoes

Nutritional Info || Protein **2g**, Fiber **4g**, Calories **200cal**
Prep time: 30 minutes

INGREDIENTS

- 2 medium sweet potatoes, peeled and diced

- 1 tablespoon olive oil, Salt and pepper to taste

INSTRUCTIONS

1. Boil sweet potatoes until tender.

2. Mash with olive oil, salt, and pepper.

Lentil and Vegetable Stew

Nutritional Info || Protein **18g**, Fiber **12g**, Calories **300cal**

Prep time: 35 minutes

INGREDIENTS

- 1 cup cooked lentils

- Mixed vegetables (carrots, celery, onions)

- Vegetable broth, Herbs and spices (thyme, bay leaves)

INSTRUCTIONS

Simmer lentils and mixed vegetables in vegetable broth with herbs and spices.

Quinoa Salad with Chickpeas

Nutritional Info || Protein **14g**, Fiber **8g**, Calories **320cal**

Prep time: 25 minutes

INGREDIENTS

- 1/2 cup cooked quinoa

- 1/2 cup canned chickpeas, rinsed

- Cherry tomatoes, halved

- Cucumber, diced

- Feta cheese crumbles

INSTRUCTIONS

Mix cooked quinoa, chickpeas, cherry tomatoes, cucumber, and feta cheese.

Turkey and Vegetable Wrap

Nutritional Info || Protein **18g**, Fiber **6g**, Calories **280cal**
Prep time: 15 minutes

INGREDIENTS

- Whole-grain wrap

- Sliced turkey breast

- Hummus,

-Sliced cucumber and bell peppers

INSTRUCTIONS

1. Spread hummus on the wrap, layer with turkey, cucumber, and bell peppers.

2. Roll into a wrap and slice

Brown Rice Bowl with Black Beans

Nutritional Info || Protein **12g**, Fiber **10g**, Calories **330cal**
Prep time: 20 minutes

INGREDIENTS

- 1/2 cup cooked brown rice

- 1/2 cup canned black beans, rinsed

- Salsa and guacamole for topping

- Fresh cilantro

INSTRUCTIONS

1. Combine cooked brown rice and black beans.

2. Top with salsa, guacamole, and fresh cilantro.

Lemon Herb Grilled Chicken

Roasted Salmon with Asparagus

Quinoa Stuffed Bell Peppers

Baked Chicken with Sweet Potato Mash

Shrimp and Broccoli Stir-Fry

Turkey and Vegetable Skewers

Lentil and Spinach Stuffed Mushrooms

Veggie and Chickpea Curry

Baked Cod with Tomato Salsa

Eggplant and Turkey Lasagna

Lemon Herb Grilled Chicken

Nutritional Info || Protein **30g**, Fiber **1g**, Calories **300cal**
Prep time: 30 minutes

INGREDIENTS

- 6 oz chicken breast

- Fresh lemon juice

- Mixed herbs (rosemary, thyme)

INSTRUCTIONS

1. Marinate chicken in lemon juice, herbs, and olive oil.

2. Grill until fully cooked.

Roasted Salmon with Asparagus

Nutritional Info || Protein **25g**, Fiber **4g**, Calories **350cal**
Prep time: 25 minutes

INGREDIENTS

- 6 oz salmon fillet

- Fresh lemon slices

- Asparagus spears

- Olive oil

INSTRUCTIONS

1. Place salmon and asparagus on a baking sheet.

2. Drizzle with olive oil, add lemon slices, and bake at 400°F (200°C) for 15-20 minutes.

Quinoa Stuffed Bell Peppers

Nutritional Info || Protein **20g**, Fiber **8g**, Calories **320cal**
Prep time: 40 minutes

INGREDIENTS

- Bell peppers, halved

- 1 cup cooked quinoa

- Lean ground turkey

- Diced tomatoes

- Black beans

INSTRUCTIONS

1. Cook ground turkey, mix with quinoa, diced tomatoes, and black beans.

2. Stuff bell peppers and bake at 375°F (190°C) for 25-30 minutes.

Baked Chicken with Sweet Potato Mash

Nutritional Info || Protein **25g**, Fiber **6g**, Calories **380cal**
Prep time: 45 minutes

INGREDIENTS

- 6 oz chicken thighs

- Sweet potatoes, peeled and diced

- Greek yogurt

- Garlic powder

INSTRUCTIONS

1. Bake chicken thighs until cooked.

2. Boil sweet potatoes, mash with Greek yogurt and garlic powder.

Shrimp and Broccoli Stir-Fry

Nutritional Info || Protein **22g**, Fiber **4g**, Calories **320cal**

Prep time: 30 minutes

INGREDIENTS

- 8 oz shrimp, peeled and deveined

- Broccoli florets

- Soy sauce

- Ginger and garlic

- Brown rice

INSTRUCTIONS

1. Stir-fry shrimp and broccoli in soy sauce, ginger, and garlic.

2. Serve over cooked brown rice.

Turkey and Vegetable Skewers

Nutritional Info || Protein **22g**, Fiber **5g**, Calories **280cal**

Prep time: 35 minutes

INGREDIENTS

- Lean ground turkey

- Bell peppers, onions, cherry tomatoes

- Olive oil

- Italian seasoning

INSTRUCTIONS

1. Mix ground turkey with olive oil and Italian seasoning.

2. Thread onto skewers with vegetables and grill until cooked.

Lentil and Spinach Stuffed Mushrooms

Nutritional Info || Protein **15g**, Fiber **8g**, Calories **240cal**

Prep time: 30 minutes

INGREDIENTS

- Portobello mushrooms, stemmed

- Cooked lentils

- Chopped spinach

- Feta cheese

INSTRUCTIONS

1. Mix lentils, chopped spinach, and feta cheese.

2. Stuff mushrooms and bake at 375°F (190°C) for 20 minutes.

Veggie and Chickpea Curry

Nutritional Info || Protein **12g**, Fiber **10g**, Calories **340cal**

Prep time: 40 minutes

INGREDIENTS

- Mixed vegetables (carrots, bell peppers, peas)

- Chickpeas

- Coconut milk

- Curry spices

- Brown rice

INSTRUCTIONS

1. Simmer mixed vegetables and chickpeas in coconut milk with curry spices.

2. Serve over cooked brown rice.

Baked Cod with Tomato Salsa

Nutritional Info || Protein **30g**, Fiber **3g**, Calories **280cal**
Prep time: 25 minutes

INGREDIENTS

- 6 oz cod fillet

- Diced tomatoes

- Red onion, diced

- Fresh cilantro

INSTRUCTIONS

1. Place cod on a baking sheet.

2. Top with a mixture of diced tomatoes, red onion, and fresh cilantro.

3. Bake at 375°F (190°C) for 20 minutes.

Eggplant and Turkey Lasagna

Nutritional Info || Protein **25g**, Fiber **6g**, Calories **350cal**
Prep time: 50 minutes

INGREDIENTS

- Eggplant, sliced

- Lean ground turkey

- Tomato sauce

- Ricotta cheese

- Mozzarella cheese

INSTRUCTIONS

1. Grill eggplant slices.

2. Layer in a baking dish with cooked ground turkey, tomato sauce, ricotta, and mozzarella.

3. Bake at 375°F (190°C) for 30 minutes.

Delectable Desserts and Satisfying Snacks for seniors

Berry Parfait

Baked Apple Slices

Chia Seed Pudding with Mango

Banana Nut Muffins (Low-Fat)

Greek Yogurt and Berries Popsicles

Dark Chocolate-Dipped Strawberries

Almond Butter and Banana Roll-Ups

Coconut and Date Energy Bites

Pumpkin Spice Smoothie

Rice Pudding with Cinnamon

Berry Parfait

Nutritional Info || Protein **10g**, Fiber **5g**, Calories **200cal**

Prep time: 10 minutes

INGREDIENTS

- Mixed berries (blueberries, strawberries, raspberries)

- Greek yogurt

- Granola

- Honey (optional)

INSTRUCTIONS

1. Layer Greek yogurt, mixed berries, and granola in a glass.

2. Drizzle with honey if desired.

Baked Apple Slices

Nutritional Info || Protein **3g**, Fiber **5g**, Calories **150cal**

Prep time: 20 minutes

INGREDIENTS

- Apple slices

- Cinnamon

- Walnuts, chopped

- Greek yogurt (optional)

INSTRUCTIONS

1. Toss apple slices with cinnamon and chopped walnuts.

2. Bake at 375°F (190°C) for 15-20 minutes.

3. Serve with a dollop of Greek yogurt if desired.

Chia Seed Pudding with Mango

Nutritional Info || Protein **5g**, Fiber **8g**, Calories **180cal**

Prep time: 5 minutes

INGREDIENTS

- Chia seeds

- Almond milk

- Mango cubes

- Shredded coconut

INSTRUCTIONS

1. Mix chia seeds and almond milk, refrigerate overnight.

2. Top with mango cubes and shredded coconut.

Banana Nut Muffins

Nutritional Info || Protein **3g**, Fiber **2g**, Calories **120cal (per muffin)**

Prep time: 25 minutes

INGREDIENTS

- Ripe bananas, mashed

- Whole wheat flour

- Chopped walnuts

- Greek yogurt

INSTRUCTIONS

1. Mix mashed bananas, whole wheat flour, chopped walnuts, and Greek yogurt.

2. Spoon into muffin cups and bake at 350°F (175°C) for 20-25 minutes.

Greek Yogurt and Berries Popsicles

Nutritional Info || Protein **6g**, Fiber **2g**, Calories **100cal**

Prep time: 15 minutes (plus freezing time)

INGREDIENTS

- Greek yogurt

- Mixed berries (strawberries, blueberries)

- Honey (optional)

INSTRUCTIONS

1. Mix Greek yogurt with berries and honey.

2. Pour into Popsicle molds and freeze.

Dark Chocolate-Dipped Strawberries

Nutritional Info || Protein **1g**, Fiber **2g**, Calories 60 (per strawberry)

Prep time: 20 minutes

INGREDIENTS

- Fresh strawberries

- Dark chocolate (70% cocoa)

- Chopped nuts (optional)

INSTRUCTIONS

1. Melt dark chocolate.

2. Dip strawberries into melted chocolate, sprinkle with chopped nuts.

Almond Butter and Banana Roll-Ups

Nutritional Info || Protein **5g**, Fiber **4g**, Calories **180cal**

Prep time: 10 minutes

INGREDIENTS

- Whole-grain tortilla

- Almond butter

- Sliced bananas

INSTRUCTIONS

1. Spread almond butter on a tortilla, place banana slices, and roll up.

2. Slice into bite-sized pieces.

Coconut and Date Energy Bites

Nutritional Info || Protein **2g**, Fiber **3g**, Calories 120 (per energy bite)

Prep time: 15 minutes

INGREDIENTS

- Dates, pitted

- Almonds

- Shredded coconut

- Vanilla extract

INSTRUCTIONS

1. Blend dates almonds, shredded coconut, and vanilla extract in a food processor.

2. Roll into small energy bites.

Pumpkin Spice Smoothie

Nutritional Info || Protein **3g**, Fiber **5g**, Calories **150cal**

Prep time: 5 minutes

INGREDIENTS

- Canned pumpkin puree

- Almond milk

- Banana

- Pumpkin spice

INSTRUCTIONS

Blend pumpkin puree, almond milk, banana, and pumpkin spice until smooth.

Rice Pudding with Cinnamon

Nutritional Info || Protein **4g**, Fiber **3g**, Calories **200cal**

Prep time: 20 minutes

INGREDIENTS

- Cooked brown rice

- Almond milk

- Maple syrup

- Cinnamon

INSTRUCTIONS

Simmer cooked brown rice in almond milk, maple syrup, and cinnamon until creamy.

HERE IS YOUR BONUS:

21-Day meal plan to get you started with the NO GALLBLADDER DIET. All recipes and instructions for preparing them have been discussed in the guide.

Day 1:

- Breakfast: Oatmeal Delight

- Lunch: Grilled Chicken Salad

- Dinner: Lemon Herb Grilled Chicken

- Snack/Dessert: Berry Parfait

Day 2:

- Breakfast: Egg White Veggie Scramble

- Lunch: Quinoa and Vegetable Bowl

- Dinner: Roasted Salmon with Asparagus

- Snack/Dessert: Baked Apple Slices

Day 3:

- Breakfast: Smoothie Bliss

- Lunch: Vegetable Soup with Whole Grain Crackers

- Dinner: Quinoa Stuffed Bell Peppers

- Snack/Dessert: Chia Seed Pudding with Mango

Day 4:

- Breakfast: Greek Yogurt Parfait

- Lunch: Baked Chicken with Sweet Potato Mash

- Dinner: Shrimp and Broccoli Stir-Fry

- Snack/Dessert: Banana Nut Muffins (Low-Fat)

Day 5:

- Breakfast: Avocado Toast with Poached Egg

- Lunch: Lentil and Vegetable Stew

- Dinner: Turkey and Vegetable Skewers

- Snack/Dessert: Greek Yogurt and Berries Popsicles

Day 6:

- Breakfast: Chia Seed Pudding

- Lunch: Quinoa Salad with Chickpeas

-Dinner: Baked Cod with Tomato Salsa

-Snack/Dessert: Dark Chocolate-Dipped Strawberries

Day 7:

- Breakfast: Blueberry Almond Overnight Oats

- Lunch: Turkey and Vegetable Wrap

- Dinner: Eggplant and Turkey Lasagna

- Snack/Dessert: Almond Butter and Banana Roll-Ups

Day 8:

- Breakfast: Banana Nut Muffins (Low-Fat)

- Lunch: Brown Rice Bowl with Black Beans

- Dinner: Lentil and Spinach Stuffed Mushrooms

- Snack/Dessert: Coconut and Date Energy Bites

Certainly! Let's continue with the meal plan for the next two weeks:

Day 9:

- Breakfast: Raspberry Almond Smoothie Bowl

- Lunch: Turkey and Vegetable Wrap

- Dinner: Quinoa Stuffed Bell Peppers

- Snack/Dessert: Greek Yogurt and Berries Popsicles

Day 10:

- Breakfast: Chia Seed Pudding with Mango

- Lunch: Veggie and Feta Frittata

- Dinner: Baked Salmon with Asparagus

- Snack/Dessert: Dark Chocolate-Dipped Strawberries

Day 11:

- Breakfast: Banana Nut Muffins (Low-Fat)

-Lunch: Greek Yogurt Parfait

- Dinner: Veggie and Chickpea Curry

- Snack/Dessert: Pumpkin Spice Smoothie

Day 12:

- Breakfast: Avocado Toast with Poached Egg

- Lunch: Quinoa Salad with Chickpeas

- Dinner: Lentil and Vegetable Stew

- Snack/Dessert: Coconut and Date Energy Bites

Day 12:

- Breakfast: Blueberry Almond Overnight Oats

- Lunch: Lentil and Spinach Stuffed Mushrooms

- Dinner: Grilled Chicken Salad

- Snack/Dessert: Baked Apple Slices

Day 13:

- Breakfast: Smoothie Bliss

- Lunch: Turkey and Vegetable Skewers

- Dinner: Lemon Herb Grilled Chicken

- Snack/Dessert: Rice Pudding with Cinnamon

Day 14:

- Breakfast: Oatmeal Delight

- Lunch: Baked Chicken with Sweet Potato Mash

- Dinner: Shrimp and Broccoli Stir-Fry

- Snack/Dessert: Almond Butter and Banana Roll-Ups

Day 15:

- Breakfast: Egg White Veggie Scramble

- Lunch: Brown Rice Bowl with Black Beans

- Dinner: Baked Cod with Tomato Salsa

- Snack/Dessert: Berry Parfait

Day 16:

- Breakfast: Greek Yogurt Parfait

- Lunch: Quinoa and Vegetable Bowl

- Dinner: Roasted Salmon with Asparagus

- Snack/Dessert: Pumpkin Spice Smoothie

Day 17:

- Breakfast: Avocado Toast with Poached Egg

- Lunch: Turkey and Vegetable Wrap

- Dinner: Eggplant and Turkey Lasagna

- Snack/Dessert: Dark Chocolate-Dipped Strawberries

Day 18:

- Breakfast: Banana Nut Muffins (Low-Fat)

- Lunch: Lentil and Vegetable Stew

- Dinner: Quinoa Stuffed Bell Peppers

- Snack/Dessert: Coconut and Date Energy Bites

Day 19:

- Breakfast: Blueberry Almond Overnight Oats

- Lunch: Veggie and Feta Frittata

- Dinner: Baked Salmon with Asparagus

- Snack/Dessert: Greek Yogurt and Berries Popsicles

Day 20:

- Breakfast: Chia Seed Pudding with Mango

- Lunch: Quinoa Salad with Chickpeas

- Dinner: Lentil and Spinach Stuffed Mushrooms

- Snack/Dessert: Baked Apple Slices

Day 21:

- Breakfast: Smoothie Bliss

- Lunch: Turkey and Vegetable Skewers

- Dinner: Lemon Herb Grilled Chicken

- Snack/Dessert: Rice Pudding with Cinnamon

Conclusion

In conclusion, this book has provided a comprehensive guide for seniors navigating the journey of a no gallbladder diet. Let's recap some key points and offer valuable tips to ensure long-term success and well-being.

Throughout these pages, we've emphasized the importance of embracing a diverse range of nutrient-rich foods. A diet rich in fruits, vegetables, lean proteins, and whole grains not only supports overall health but also assists in managing the unique challenges faced after gallbladder removal. Portion control, the inclusion of healthy fats, and prioritizing sources of lean protein have been highlighted as essential components of a balanced diet tailored for seniors.

Hydration remains a crucial aspect of daily life, as seniors are more prone to dehydration. Choosing whole, minimally processed foods and limiting sodium intake contributes to better cardiovascular health. The incorporation of colorful fruits and vegetables ensures a spectrum of essential vitamins and minerals, promoting optimal well-being.

Meal timing and establishing a regular eating routine have been discussed as strategies to enhance digestion and support overall health. Encouraging social interactions during meals not only creates enjoyable dining experiences but also contributes to emotional well-being, a vital aspect of senior health.

As you embark on this journey, it's important to adapt to changing needs and stay flexible with your dietary choices. Personal preferences, cultural considerations, and individual tastes should always be taken into account. Regular consultations with healthcare professionals, including dietitians, can provide personalized guidance, ensuring your diet aligns with your specific health conditions and nutritional requirements.

Lastly, let me offer words of encouragement for your long-term success. Embracing a no gallbladder diet may present challenges, but with dedication and the right knowledge, you are well-equipped to lead a healthy and fulfilling life. Celebrate the small victories, listen to your body, and remember that every positive choice contributes to your overall well-being.

May this book serve as a valuable companion on your journey towards optimal health after gallbladder removal. Here's to your continued success, vitality, and the joy of savoring every moment of life.

Meal planner journal

Dates

	BREAKFAST	LUNCH	DINNER	SNACKS
MON				
TUE				
WED				
THU				
FRI				
SAT				
SUN				

Shopping list

Note

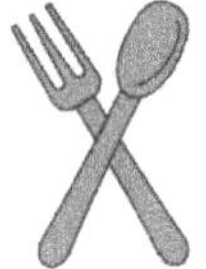

Meal planner journal

Dates

	BREAKFAST	LUNCH	DINNER	SNACKS
MON				
TUE				
WED				
THU				
FRI				
SAT				
SUN				

Shopping list

Note

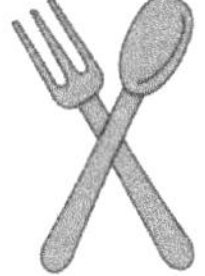

Meal planner journal

| | Dates |

	BREAKFAST	LUNCH	DINNER	SNACKS
MON				
TUE				
WED				
THU				
FRI				
SAT				
SUN				

Shopping list

Note

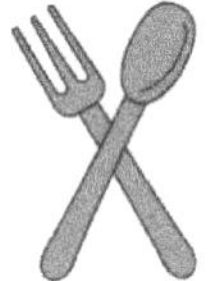

Meal planner journal

Dates

	BREAKFAST	LUNCH	DINNER	SNACKS
MON				
TUE				
WED				
THU				
FRI				
SAT				
SUN				

Shopping list

Note

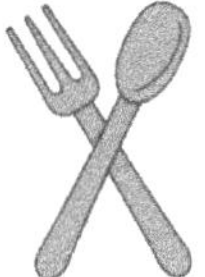

Meal planner journal

Dates

	BREAKFAST	LUNCH	DINNER	SNACKS
MON				
TUE				
WED				
THU				
FRI				
SAT				
SUN				

Shopping list

Note

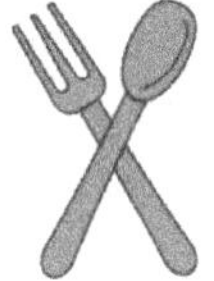

Meal planner journal

Dates

	BREAKFAST	LUNCH	DINNER	SNACKS
MON				
TUE				
WED				
THU				
FRI				
SAT				
SUN				

Shopping list

Note

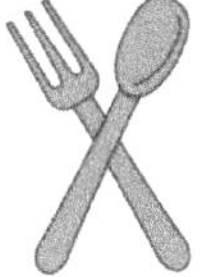

Meal planner journal

Dates

	BREAKFAST	LUNCH	DINNER	SNACKS
MON				
TUE				
WED				
THU				
FRI				
SAT				
SUN				

Shopping list

Note

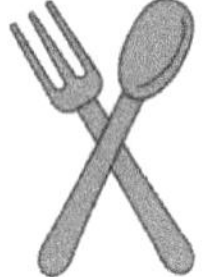

Meal planner journal

Dates

	BREAKFAST	LUNCH	DINNER	SNACKS
MON				
TUE				
WED				
THU				
FRI				
SAT				
SUN				

Shopping list

Note

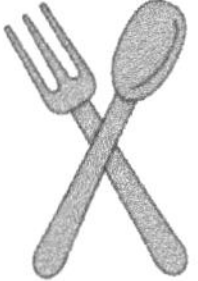

Meal planner journal

Dates

	BREAKFAST	LUNCH	DINNER	SNACKS
MON				
TUE				
WED				
THU				
FRI				
SAT				
SUN				

Shopping list

Note

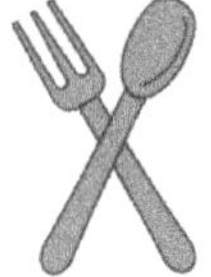

Meal planner journal

Dates

	BREAKFAST	LUNCH	DINNER	SNACKS
MON				
TUE				
WED				
THU				
FRI				
SAT				
SUN				

Shopping list

Note

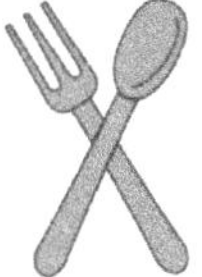

Meal planner journal

Dates

	BREAKFAST	LUNCH	DINNER	SNACKS
MON				
TUE				
WED				
THU				
FRI				
SAT				
SUN				

Shopping list

Note

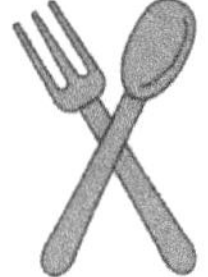

Meal planner journal

Dates

	BREAKFAST	LUNCH	DINNER	SNACKS
MON				
TUE				
WED				
THU				
FRI				
SAT				
SUN				

Shopping list

Note

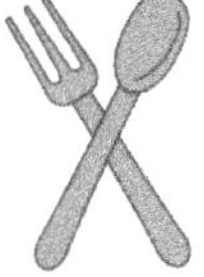

Meal planner journal

Dates

	BREAKFAST	LUNCH	DINNER	SNACKS
MON				
TUE				
WED				
THU				
FRI				
SAT				
SUN				

Shopping list

____
____
____
____
____

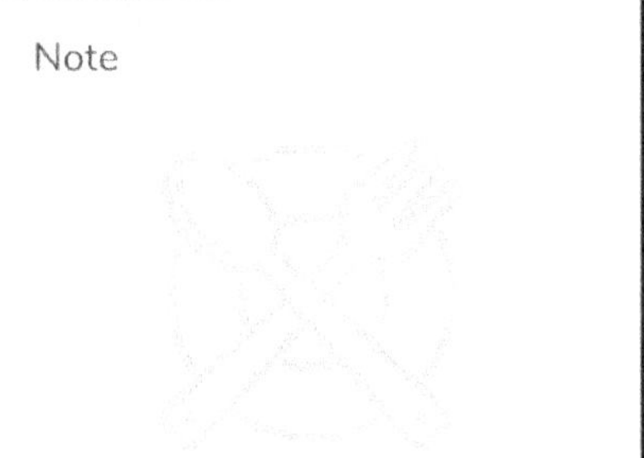

Note

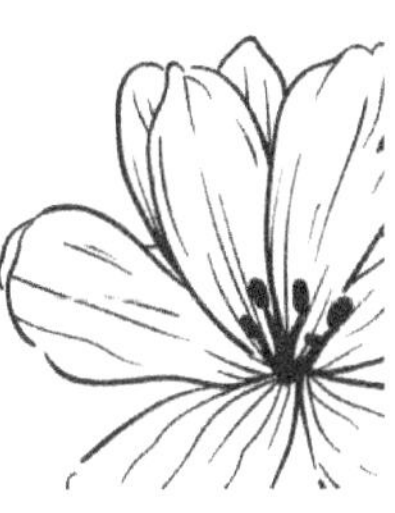

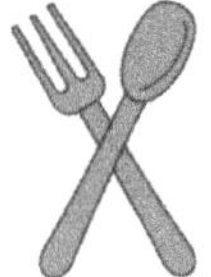 # *Meal planner journal*

Dates

	BREAKFAST	LUNCH	DINNER	SNACKS
MON				
TUE				
WED				
THU				
FRI				
SAT				
SUN				

Shopping list

Note

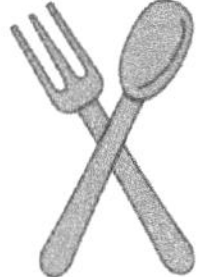

Meal planner journal

Dates

	BREAKFAST	LUNCH	DINNER	SNACKS
MON				
TUE				
WED				
THU				
FRI				
SAT				
SUN				

Shopping list

Note

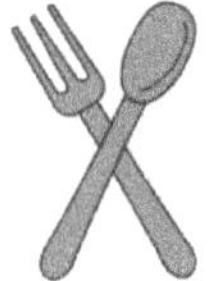

Meal planner journal

Dates

	BREAKFAST	LUNCH	DINNER	SNACKS
MON				
TUE				
WED				
THU				
FRI				
SAT				
SUN				

Shopping list

Note

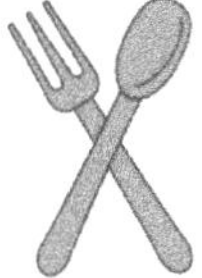

Meal planner journal

Dates

	BREAKFAST	LUNCH	DINNER	SNACKS
MON				
TUE				
WED				
THU				
FRI				
SAT				
SUN				

Shopping list

Note

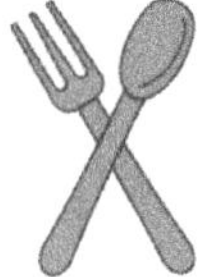

Meal planner journal

Dates

	BREAKFAST	LUNCH	DINNER	SNACKS
MON				
TUE				
WED				
THU				
FRI				
SAT				
SUN				

Shopping list

Note

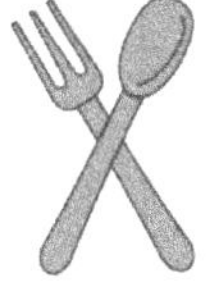

Meal planner journal

Dates

	BREAKFAST	LUNCH	DINNER	SNACKS
MON				
TUE				
WED				
THU				
FRI				
SAT				
SUN				

Shopping list

Note

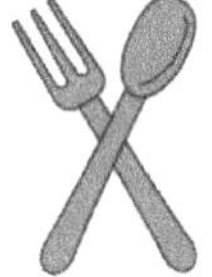

Meal planner journal

Dates

	BREAKFAST	LUNCH	DINNER	SNACKS
MON				
TUE				
WED				
THU				
FRI				
SAT				
SUN				

Shopping list

Note

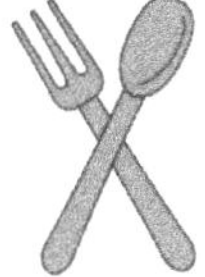

Meal planner journal

Dates

	BREAKFAST	LUNCH	DINNER	SNACKS
MON				
TUE				
WED				
THU				
FRI				
SAT				
SUN				

Shopping list

Note

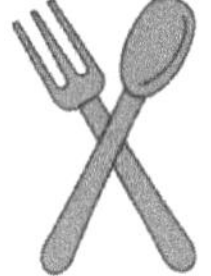

Meal planner journal

Dates

	BREAKFAST	LUNCH	DINNER	SNACKS
MON				
TUE				
WED				
THU				
FRI				
SAT				
SUN				

Shopping list

Note

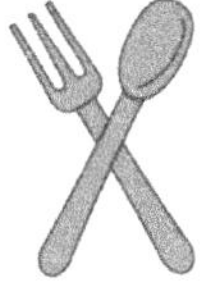

Meal planner journal

Dates

	BREAKFAST	LUNCH	DINNER	SNACKS
MON				
TUE				
WED				
THU				
FRI				
SAT				
SUN				

Shopping list

____

____

____

____

____

____

Note

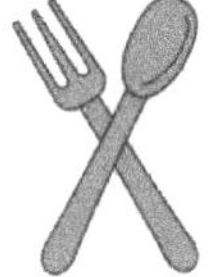

Meal planner journal

Dates

	BREAKFAST	LUNCH	DINNER	SNACKS
MON				
TUE				
WED				
THU				
FRI				
SAT				
SUN				

Shopping list

Note

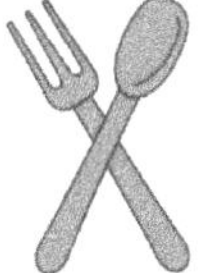

Meal planner journal

Dates

	BREAKFAST	LUNCH	DINNER	SNACKS
MON				
TUE				
WED				
THU				
FRI				
SAT				
SUN				

Shopping list

____
____
____
____
____

Note